THE ECONOMICS OF HEALTH

Keith E. Lindsey, Ph.D.

THE ECONOMICS OF HEALTH

In memory of my grandparents Leon, Helen, Mary, and Rommie.

To my mom, Shirley, and sister, Kishia, for always supporting me.

To my wife, Charlene, for allowing me to think and type at all hours of the day and night.

To my son, Keith II, who I hope through my example will grow to be an even better man than me.

Contents

Since the beginning of recorded history, health has always been in the forefront of society. The ability to protect the country's welfare started well before those words were mentioned in the United States Constitution. The successful pursuit of happiness and life cannot occur without health, and in our country, it is a well fought battle.

The United States is one of the wealthiest countries in the world, yet it lags in public health advocacy efforts. I think some of this message gets over politicized, so the real good that could be accomplished by man is often thrown to the wayside due to political pandering, partisan griping, and political posturing. It is quite obvious our nation faces a flux of challenges when it comes to health; however, most of it is based on the tenet of you can be where am I, except every citizen does not live on the same economic level, so this sadly leads to unrealistic results and demands.

This now opens a door of realistic thinking to logically surmise that a false premise can lead to a false conclusion. This was something I learned in high school mathematics, but the profound inclination of change cannot be beautifully pontificated, it is going to take people willing to stand in front of issues to be a true public advocate. We all know where the health of our country is going; the issue at hand is how to open the window of inflexibility and allow the air of common sense to flood the room.

Health, a universal, fundamental need, has become a firestorm in our country with the passage of the Affordable Care Act. The battle for equal care, affordable rates, and the insurability of individuals has been the subject of vitriol from both sides of the health argument. As people in the country rally and take sides on this issue, how many people are looking at the full economic picture the law? The importance of health as an economic factor is as equally important as being in good health in able to generate economic growth and stability.

The health of a nation compared to its peers is important because it allows us to realize how effective our dollars are being spent. Is there really a cultural, economic, and class separation or are we simply using buzz words to scare people into believing our words? The answer to this question could be as difficult as the sphinx presenting its riddle to wayward travelers, devouring them if they could not answer the riddle correctly.

The concept of this book is not to take a partisan side on this issue because our health does not subscribe to a particular political thought or agenda. The issue of health should not be caught up in the emotional aspects of people, but to take the middle of the road to ascertain how change can be effective when we do not blur the lines of communication. The discussion about health should not be regulated to stifle communication, but should open avenues of dialogue to listen and reflect about the multiple factors that could affect health in the community. When this happens, we will be getting to yes; we will become a unified force to improve the health of our great nation.

We must be willing use our collective knowledge to increase and advance health on a national and local level. At some point in this continuing discussion, I firmly believe common sense and practicality will rule the day over politics and separatism. In our time, we should not see people die from preventable diseases, yet this is the choice they make by their lifestyle decisions.

Progressive, socialist, conservative, tea party, libertarian, and people all across the vast spectrum of religion have one thing in common; our lives are linear, and having good health is vital to ensuring the years we have are lived to its fullest. Therefore, health is not simply an issue for the poor or minorities, it is a national issue with global ramifications. Our health does not respond to personal or partisan bickering; however, it does tell us when we are not doing right to our bodies and the telling effects it has on both person and society.

Health is an interesting topic because it can be seen through different prisms; therefore, it evokes varying expressions of thoughts, attitudes, behaviors, and beliefs. It portrays a life of its own through the eyes of employers, employees, unemployed, underemployed, and those who receive public assistance. Not only does it portray life, but it holds a different level of value when taken into consideration by various groups.

Health also takes on the form of money when viewed from the eyes of a practitioner, insurance companies, employers, and employees. The questions of benefits versus payments, copayments, deductibles, and maintaining a standard level of care becomes quite a concern. There are questions of abuse, fraud, mismanagement, gouging, and whether the system is "pricing out" the cost of health that raise concerns because the answers are not always forthcoming by those in leadership.

I hope you enjoy reading my opinion on state of health in the United States. I hope the information presented will hopefully increase and expand our thinking about health, and how a dollar price cannot be attributed to our health because it is priceless. This book will provide some very interesting talking points about health services and delivery versus the price paid to maintain our current status quo.

Chapter 1: Health in the United States

Health has always been an item of concern and interest in the United States. From the beginning of this country to the present day, we have been focused on protecting the overall health of the country and its citizens through the passage laws and ordinances. Most of the statutes are state specific; however, there are others that set federal standards for environmental controls. These laws include the Clean Water Act, Clean Air Act, Health Insurance Portability and Accountability Act (HIPAA), Ryan White CARE Act, Comprehensive Environmental Response, Compensation, and Liability Act (CERCLA), and Resource Conservation and Recovery Act (RCRA).

These laws were put into place to ensure the country would not jeopardize the present and future state of health of the general population. Not many would disagree with the assessment of having policies to ensure we have safe water to drink, clean air to breath, good hygienic principles, immunization schedules, and other practices we often take for granted. The proper use of regulatory oversight is good for the well-being of the nation to protect us from ourselves.

Poor health is often attributed to third world and undeveloped countries. However, the Commonwealth Fund ranked the United States last for performance among 11 industrialized nations in a 2014 report. This would be inconceivable for most people in the health and medical field, but this takes into consideration the United States ranked number one in healthcare expense.

The answer to this question should be of great interest to the citizens of this country because are we really receiving quality care for the money being invested into the system? Could it be possible to believe we the consumers are the recipients of a poor product? Could it be our healthcare system, though advanced, still falls behind our world peers in terms of producing better health outcomes? Could it be theorized that the citizens of these countries care more about their health than the United States? Even though these are hypothetical questions that are sure to raise a rigorous debate, the harsh reality is we have the answers to these questions. However, the answers will most certainly not be popular, but a little debate can go a long way in reforming the healthcare system.

A World Perspective

When considering the overall health of the nation, it is always good to realize how each segment of the population is faring. The life expectancy for females and males in the United States is 81 years and 76 years respectively; however, the average expectancy of 78.7 years ranked 26 out of 40 developed countries when comparing the life expectancy of individuals.

In continuing the review of health among the United States population, it was further categorized to ascertain the health of the population by race and specific health ailments. Fifty-one percent of the population has been diagnosed with hypertension. In white males and females the rate is 58.7% and 42.8%, and in black males and females the rate is 68.9% and 46.8%. The higher numbers illustrate the disparity between races; however, there are cultural and other dynamics that have not been factored in these percentages.

Chronic Diseases

The top ten chronic conditions in the United States are:

1. Cardiovascular Disease

2. Hypertension

3. Stroke

4. Diabetes

5. Cancer

6. Arthritis

7. Hepatitis

8. Chronic Obstructive Pulmonary Disease (COPD)

9. Asthma

10. Kidneys

In 2012, 85.6% percent of the population had at least one chronic condition. In addition, the percentages of chronic diseases ranked very different across racial lines in regards to how many people in the population were afflicted with chronic diseases.

	0-1	2-3	4+
Black	71.7%	22.6%	5.8%
White	77.0%	18.9%	4.1%
Asian	82.5%	15.0%	2.4%
Hispanic	79.4%	16.4%	4.2%
Mexican	80.0%	16.2%	3.8%

African-Americans have the highest percentage of multiple chronic diseases in comparison to other races; however, they have the lowest percentage of having only one chronic disease. Conversely, Asians are more likely to have at least one chronic disease, but their numbers decreases significantly in regards to having multiple chronic diseases.

From this, it would appear culture does factor into health consciousness of a population.

Health Insurance Coverage

In light of this information, 15.8% of the population does not have health insurance coverage, and the states uninsured percentage ranges from 4.3% to 24.3%. Here a list ranking the states with the highest percentage of uninsured citizens in 2012:

1. Texas (24.3%)

2. Nevada (22.5%)

3. New Mexico (21.0%)

4. Florida (20.7%)

5. Louisiana (19.7%)

6. Georgia (19.3%)

7. California (19.0%)

8. Alaska (18.4%)

9. Arizona (18.2%)

10. Montana (18.2%)

Here is a ranking of the states with the lowest percentage of uninsured citizens in 2012:

1. Massachusetts (4.3%)

2. Hawaii (7.8%)

3. Vermont (8.3%)

4. Minnesota (9.1%)

5. Connecticut (9.3%)

6. Maine (9.6%)

7. District of Columbia (9.7%)

8. Wisconsin (9.8%)

9. Delaware (10.7%)

10. Indiana (10.8%)

The conversion of these percentages to numbers would highlight a staggering number of people who are without insurance. In review of the states with the highest percentage, some rank in the top ten percent of the United States population. Also, the highest percentages of these people reside in the Southwestern (4 states) and Southern (3 states) regions of the United States. Conversely, the lowest percentages are found in the Northeastern (4 states) and Midwestern (3 states) regions of the United States. It would be prudent to mention that many of these states have lower population densities and a lower total income, yet the majority of their citizens are insured.

The insurance coverage of individuals can be through the private market or through public exchanges. In 2012, the breakdown of percentages of citizens by race that were insured through private health exchanges was as followed:

White-64.8%

Black-45.8%

American Indian-34.9%

Asian-67.6%

Hispanic/Latino-36.7%

The majority of the minority populations does not have insurance through a private provider that could indicate they are not employed, cannot afford the insurance, or rely on government assistance to provide their healthcare needs. By geographic location, the South has the lowest percentage of private coverage at 57.3% versus the highest percentage found in the Midwest at 68.4%.

Quality versus Quantity

The ability to obtain quality healthcare is dependent upon who wants to insure the individual, along with the perceived risks of insuring them. The quality of care issue is a subplot to how should this care be paid for, whether it should be mandated, or what a person should do to ensure their basic healthcare needs are being met. These are the questions being placed in the minds of citizens, politicians, media and think groups. The answers to these health questions are found by reviewing the numbers refute blind allegations, biased thinking, and information not based on science.

Even though numbers can sometimes be skewed towards a thought, this one thing is undeniable, America for all its worth falls way behind the curve when it comes to having a healthy society. This is partially due economic inequality, educational levels, family structure, culture, and traditions. The solution to these questions are complicated; however, understanding these basic numbers set the table for more enhanced, quality conversations about health in the United States.

Some would argue that you cannot compare the quality and quantity of health in other countries because care in the United States is superior. I would counter this argument with a conversation I had with an old college friend who lives and works in another country. He needed to have two crowns and fillings that were performed by the local dentist; the total price for the procedure was less than one hundred dollars.

Now, the dentist charged my friend more because he was a "rich American". If I were to have the same procedures performed, my out of pocket cost would total over $1,000 and that is with the insurance company paying at least half of the costs. In analysis of both situations, assuming the dentist is utilizing the same materials, dental equipment, and procedures, who is getting the better cost for his care? My friend was more than satisfied with the work and remarked about how having the same procedure performed in the current system would have taken him to the cleaners.

The Burden of Health

What is the overall burden for health in the United States? What is the overarching burden of health? What are the telltale factors that inhibit the adoption of more healthy lifestyles? One only has to observe the habits of a population that would quickly aid you in understanding why their health is not improving at the rate we would desire. The first step starts with reviewing the economic factors that deter good health and then talk about the amalgamation of culture that further stratifies the population.

Health, like beauty, is in the eye of the beholder. Now the biggest question in the room can become a little smaller with increasing education, lifestyle evaluations, and their personal decisions that influence health. Most of those decisions also lie with the community in which they reside.

Many Americans live in food deserts, in either rural or urban designations, where there is not affordable, nutritious food within a 10 mile or 1 mile driving radius, respectively, of their residences. This designation affects almost 2.5 million Americans, and can be affiliated with lower economics, higher food prices, lower quality foods, and the need for reliable transportation.

Our health is influenced by various factors such as economics, transportation, and education. Can our nation's health be improved? I truly believe it can; however, the solution starts in the local community and works itself outward in a concentric circle.

The larger community could aid in evolving an individual's environment because local actions drive state and national reactions. This is the challenge of health in the United States; taking a national health issue and transforming it into a local topic of conversation for creating change. This is important because the United States ranks in the bottom of industrialized nations in regards to the quality of care.

Health for All?

We face an assault from all sides. Just recently, we heard about the water problem in Flint, Michigan. How could any sane person justify a town consuming water with high levels of bacteria, other microorganisms, and lead? The questions in the room are pointing to those responsible in an attempt to ascertain their knowledge of the problem, and why would they choose to follow this questionable course of action. The economics of communities drive the health message and it does cause systemic problems in the overall health of communities.

In general, most people select homes based on education, crime rates, access to medical care, neighborhood dynamics, and other parameters. However, poorer community have fewer of these resources and inadequate schools, so money does not flow into the community, which hinders economic growth and development. Health outcomes are directly impacted by this and any survey of neighborhoods around the United States will illustrate this phenomenon.

The burning question surrounding health is when will people realize health is a money grab? The economics of your health are based on numbers, risk, and cost. Have you ever taken notice of the number of hospitals and clinics in your community? Have you ever wondered why certain areas seem to have the lion's share of medical resources? The easiest answer is to follow the money. It is common knowledge that more affluent neighborhoods have better access to care. When you have time, do a search of hospitals by your zip code. The truth will become obvious when you discover your health is truly dictated by your community's economic status.

The Cost of Health

There are many discussions concerning the cost of healthcare; however, before an analysis of health can be given, one must take into consideration what people think about healthcare. The opinions of healthcare and the healthcare system are not generalized according to need, there are often placed into political stances, which doesn't always attribute to open dialogue for the free exchange of information and thoughts. Either way, the comments range from support and advocacy, to condemnation of the Affordable Care Act, which some believe is the leading factor in the detriment of our current healthcare system.

In 2012, the United States allocated 17.6% of its gross domestic product (GDP) to healthcare, which is two and a half times more than any other industrialized nation according to the Organization for Economic Co-operation and Development (OECD). Here are a few more numbers and quick facts about the economic cost of healthcare:

- The United States spends 2.1 trillion dollars on health care. Drug costs represent 98 billion dollars, and Health administration costs represent 91 billion dollars.

- The U.S. spent $8,233 on health per person in 2010. The average spending on health care among the other 33 developed OECD countries was $3,268 per person.

- Spending on almost every area of healthcare is higher in the United States than in other countries.

- A large amount of higher overall hospital spending in the United States can be explained by those services costing more. The average price of service in the United States is 85% higher than the average in other OECD countries.

- A hospital stay in the United States costs over $18,000 on average. Across OECD countries, the average cost of a hospital stay is about one-third that of the U.S., at $6,200.

- **The US spends more on health care than the next 10 biggest spenders combined: Japan, Germany, France, China, the U.K., Italy, Canada, Brazil, Spain, and Australia.**

- U.S. physicians receive a higher income than physicians in other countries.

- The U.S. uses more expensive diagnostic procedures.

- Patients ask for more tests and services out of comfort not because they are medically necessary.

The outward attention of cost is often mitigated with the need to have access to care. The continued rising cost of medicine and healthcare is alarming because with the increase in technology and other medical breakthroughs, one would expect the cost to decrease; however the opposite effect is taking place.

Health Abroad

Even though the United States spends 17.6% of its GDP on healthcare expenditures; however, how are healthcare expenditures expressed in other industrialized nations. The countries of Norway, the Netherlands, and Switzerland are the next highest spenders of healthcare dollars, yet they all spent at least $3,000 less per person. France and Japan demonstrate that it is possible to have a cost-containment system while simultaneously paying their physicians using similar tools to those used in the U.S.

Here are a few key items of interest when comparing the healthcare mandates of these OECD countries to the United States:

1. They use a common fee schedule so the hospitals, doctors, and health services are paid similar rates for most of the patients they see.

2. In Sweden, all drug prescribing is done electronically.

3. Many OECD countries use strong regulations to set prices that hospitals can charge for different services, and some of them even set budgets for how much hospitals can spend.

4. Switzerland provides a ranking of hospital services from most to least expensive. Groups of insurers and hospitals across different regions then use the ranking to negotiate what prices they ought to pay.

Service vs Cost

In the U.S., how much a health care service provider gets paid depends on the kind of insurance a patient possesses. This means health care servicers can choose patients who have an insurance policy that pays them more generously than other patients who have lower-paying insurers, such as Medicaid. In comparison, the payment rates in the United States are less flexible. They are often statutory and Medicare cannot change the rates without approval by Congress. This makes the system very inflexible for cost containment.

OECD countries are more responsive to the cost of healthcare. They are flexible in responding if they think certain costs are exceeding what has been budgeted. In Japan, if spending in a specific area seems to be growing faster than projected, they lower fees for that area. In France, an organization called The French National Health Insurance Fund for Salaried Worker (CNMATS)* closely monitors spending across all kinds of services. If they see a particular area is growing faster than they expected, they can intervene by lowering the price for that service.

Health or Wealth

The World Health Organization stated the United States had 700,000 families go bankrupt trying to pay for insurance; has fewer doctors and nurses in comparison to peer countries; and possess a high infant mortality rate. At the same time, in 2009, the Department for Health and Human Services stated insurance companies made 12 billion dollars in profit. The Agency for Healthcare Research and Quality stated care for minorities is poorer, so there is an issue trying to improve the overall health for all people in this country. The challenge for the nation and its citizens is how to balance the ballooning cost of healthcare and maintain their health.

---

* English for Caisse nationale de l'assurance maladie des travailleurs salariés

I had a few interesting conversations with friends from various economic and political persuasions about the state of the health in the United States. Without hesitation, they all exclaimed how can a country of this magnitude, world stature, and economic power not have the ability to ensure a person can visit the doctor when they are sick. They then took different philosophical reasons as to why and how this could occur; however, the end result was they were concerned about their fellow man. They also wondered about how the money we spend abroad could be reinvested to bolster the quality of life in the United States.

It most certainly points towards a more troubled future, one glummer than exhorted by our nation's leaders. However, there is always a ray of hope in every cloud, and this is the ability for people to finally say enough is enough and for our leaders to start to have a genuine, vested interest in their future.

Chapter Two: Health and Culture

It is not uncommon to hear the phrase "American culture", but how many can definitely state what exactly does this culture contain? Usually when one thinks of culture, the mind gravitates towards shared rituals and practices that result in a common denominator of thought and focus. However, in America, this term is an oxymoron because America does not have a culture per se. Some may disagree with this statement, so please allow me the space to expand on this thought.

From an anthropological standpoint, culture is defined as a way of living that is built up and passed down to subsequent generations of people. Therefore, the challenge to define culture cannot be painted with a broad stroke, but with several small strokes due to the large number of ethnicities that comprise America. Also, the very definition would suggest some form of equality among its denizens, so here within lies another issue to be addressed.

America is a multicultural nation that has a myriad of ways to promote and sustain various proposals for health, economics, and overall personal viability. When we define culture, we assume we have a commonality of dress, language, social habits, communication, and eating styles. We also assume that every person has been integrated into this culture and share the same beliefs and standards.

Ethnicities

We would do better to state the American culture is comprised of several ethnicities that makes the country function as a whole. The denizens in this picture should focus more on the ethnic side than the cultural side because each individual can openly relate with one or more groups of people. Quite simply, it is the acknowledgement of ethnicities that unite us and culture seeks to separate us based on our ethnical configuration. It is similar to making the sun be representative of culture and the planets represent ethnicity. We know the sun provides universal warmth and light, but the degree and intensity of its effects depends on the planet's distance from the sun.

Another mistake is overly interchanging these words to mean that every person who resides in America has been freely accepted to a place at the table called society. This line of thinking actually moves people to accept acculturation, a term that means individuals give up their way of living to adapt to the traits of another. This might also lead to the premise there is not a true blending of culture and ethnicities, just a desire to have one become the most dominant. This directly impacts the relationship of

19

community building because acculturation often precedes assimilation. Now how does this directly affect health?

Defining Health

Health is defined as a state of overall health and not merely the absence of disease. Health, like beauty, resides in the eye of the beholder. The most important questions to ask is how does health affected by ethnicity and how willing are we to accept we are engaged in an active ethnical and cultural war in America.

Every person has pride in their origins and we are stronger and better as a nation to not disregard these differences, but to embrace them and cultivate open lines of dialogue and communication. This could provide the space to not hate or fear that which is unknown, but to use the vacuum of silence to move dialogue about health forward.

Culture and tradition play a significant role in the health of an individual. Many times, people tend to overlook the 'people factor' in health because it is often the elephant in the room. Even more, it is the one fact people hate to acknowledge due to the fact it could create an atmosphere of uncomfortable conversation about their personal life. Through my experiences I have found this area to be the most uncomfortable conversation to have because it requires a real in-depth discussion about what fuels and motivates them.

The realization of self is a very interesting topic of conversation in many situations because learning about health is personal. When retrospectively looking at life, one could see how their environment aided in shaping their thoughts, actions, and attitudes towards health. Many will often start out by explaining about what they ate as children and how this has followed them through life. We are quick to point out environmental issues that lead to unhealthy outcomes, but we still need to take an introspective view into how culture and tradition also play an active role in the decision making process.

Culture Redefined

I am going to repeat a statement that I plan to discussion in the following pages, *THERE IS NO SUCH THING AS AMERICAN CULTURE.* This is the biggest, hypocritical statement applied to generalizing the status of people in this country in an attempt to sterilize an individual's cultural identity. We have ethnic cultures and identities based on how we were raised and our cultural background. Culture, according to Merriam-Webster, has three distinct meanings;

21

1. The beliefs, customs, arts, etc., of a particular society, group, place, or time

2. A particular society that has its own beliefs, ways of life, art, etc.

3. The integrated pattern of human knowledge, belief, and behavior that depends upon the capacity for learning and transmitting knowledge to succeeding generations.

So in this respect, the racial and ethnic composition of the United States would make it virtually impossible to have a universal culture. In the same light, every race has different ethnic features and traditions. From a health perspective, every individual is a product of their individual upbringing, present decisions, and present views on health. For most, it is a reflection on what was done as a child, and these thoughts are passed down to subsequent generations, akin to having a family recipe that has been passed down through the family.

Stereotypes

Culture often opens us up to stereotypes and generalizations because populations truly misunderstand the word culture and often interchanges it with ethnicity. However, ethnic is defined by Merriam-Webster as "relating to large groups of people classed according to common racial, national, tribal, religious, linguistic, or cultural origin or background." In review of the words culture and ethnic, it can be observed that ethnic takes culture into consideration; however, culture does not take ethnic backgrounds into consideration.

America is such a conglomerate of people that you cannot place everyone into comfortable blocks because it is the ultimate melting pot. I remember having a conversation with someone concerning culture in their healthcare practice. The learning about different cultures and what they would do was placed in a neat little book as a reference tool. However, people do not always fit the casual definitions and boxes that we create; it could prove to be a far more dangerous tool to use because of the possibility of increasing or enhancing stereotypes.

The next question to be answered revolves around how does health take into consideration the various ethnic and cultural beliefs of a population. For most, it is a matter of assimilation, which ultimately has the opinion that every person should seek to belong to the majority and give up what makes you unique. This can be in the form of a business's philosophy, religious belief, or society's view of health. So it is safe to say the health needs of the population should, and must, focus on the differences to order to find commonality.

Cultural Misinterpretations

Culture separates this country because of a blind misunderstanding of integration. Health subsequently becomes collateral damage in this fight because we do not understand or take the time to recognize good health is a cultural phenomenon totally based on the ethnic status of a person and their respective environment. Negative attitudes towards ethnic views results in a shutdown of the individual because you cannot articulate health unless you understand how they live and function within the boundaries of their environment.

A similar statement can also be made in regards to the overall insight of health. Too often we paint pictures of health based on demographics; however, an insufficient amount of time is given to understanding the thoughts, feelings, beliefs, and attitudes of the population in question. A perfect example of this thought can be found in the reporting of statistical data.

If a particular zip code dies from a chronic disease, does it mean every person who resides among this zip code unhealthy? Does it mean every person is doomed to die a tragic death? Does it mean the community cannot change this status? Health is not some ambiguous anomaly; it is the sum of various moving parts that must be aligned to work in an effective manner.

Culture is the tool that is used to perform this alignment because it requires sensitivity, dialogue, and communication. The creation of a health movement, spurred by the effective understanding of culture, will assist in moving the conversation forward. The ability to apply critical thinking and cause-effect approaches to the health crisis is a positive move towards positive social change.

Understanding and respecting the bridge of culture and health is one way to achieve this goal. Another way of reaching this goal is through attaining knowledge through active research and open dialogue with others to decrease the perception of health stigmas and biases. These biases and stigmas comes from the perceived perceptions people have about one another, which from a health standpoint, could result in deadly consequences. This is due to stalling the pipeline of information which prevents communities from receiving important health information that could aid them in modifying their lifestyles.

Motivating lifestyle changes through understanding culture is a foundation of health. The lack of cultural competency creates barriers to good health in populations that sometimes cannot be overcome. Many health professionals will tell you that knowing your environment and the people who exist within it is the most important part of program building, networking, community outreach, and community development.

The Health Paradigm

Now health has taken on a multicultural dimension in the administration of programs, program development, and program implementation. The next question on the table relates to how does health promotion and culture impact health in regards to prevention and intervention strategies. The words tradition, family history, and cultural identity become active barriers to health due to people having different lifestyle habits. The identity of health is now wrapped in a cultural cocoon from a barrier standpoint along with the role of religion, language, location, gender, and age. Health professionals and scholars are looking towards social ecology as a means to promote health and change lifestyles through understanding society.

In light of this social ecology, many have thought about how this could translate into effective programs that truly engage the community. This concept transcends basic family tradition and shared values; it delves in the greater psyche of people in an attempt to discover how their psychological tendencies could affect their physical health.

What is the ecological landscape of the United States? It is trending towards minorities becoming the majority; however, the healthcare system is still being underutilized by minorities in the present. Although the racial composition of the country will always stand out as a question of interest; the future of this country from an ecological view still reveals there is a long way to go as far as race relations are concerned. There are still prejudiced and racist people, there are still people who think people are inferior based on their outward appearance, and there are still factions of people who wish to return to a more "civil" time in this country's history.

The future of health in the United States is not solely based on data, even though health funding is data driven. The future lies in people being able to communicate with one another regardless of race, class, and position to effectively discuss, promote, and advance an ever changing health climate. Without this, all of the initiatives the nation could imagine and hope to implement will not serve the community. Health and culture are delicately intertwined with the future of the country hanging in the balance. The choice is quite obvious, work together to increase our health status, or be separated and die as either a direct or indirect result of our ignorance.

Chapter 3: The Affordable Care Act

The Patient Protection and Affordable Care Act (affectionately called "Obamacare") was signed into law by President Barak Obama on March 23, 2010. The act is divided into ten titles and was initially enacted in 2014. Prior to its inception, the healthcare of America has been a hot-button topic among the citizens, politicians and special interest groups through several presidential administrations. In summary, the provisions of this bill are to include the following:

1. Expanding Medicaid eligibility.

2. Subsidizing insurance premiums.

3. Providing incentives for businesses to provide health care benefits.

4. Prohibiting denial of coverage/claims based on pre-existing conditions.

5. Establishing health insurance exchanges, and support for medical research.

The costs of these provisions are offset by a variety of taxes, fees, and cost-saving measures, such as new Medicare taxes for high-income brackets, taxes on indoor tanning, improved fairness in the Medicare

Advantage program relative to traditional Medicare, and fees on medical devices and pharmaceutical companies. There is also a tax penalty for citizens who do not obtain health insurance. The bill was passed in the senate by a vote of 60-39; and was passed in the house by a vote of 219-212.

The implementation of the bill would be a gradual phase-in over a period of four years, with some bill provisions becoming effective immediately. Here is a listing of the implementation dates and their respective provisions.

The Bill Provisions

The Affordable Care Act (ACA) provided several changes to the patients, providers, drug and medical companies in regards to treatment, price, and availability. The ACA focused on patient protection, cheaper drugs, and ensuring people could obtain affordable insurance. The other part of the Act tried to reform the system to work more efficient and save money, while not sacrificing patient services. Here a few highlights, both pro and con, of the bill;

Pros

1. Members of Congress and their staff will only be offered health care plans through the exchange or plans otherwise established by the bill.

2. The Food and Drug Administration was authorized to approve generic versions of biologic drugs and grant biologics manufacturers 12 years of exclusive use before generics can be developed.

3. Adults with pre-existing conditions will be eligible to join a temporary high-risk pool, which would be superseded by the health care exchange in 2014.

4. Allow premiums to vary by age (4:1), geographic area, and family composition.

5. Limit out-of-pocket spending to $5,950 for individuals and $11,900 for families, excluding premiums.

6. Insurance companies were prohibited from imposing lifetime dollar limits on essential benefits, like hospital stays in new policies issued.

7. Dependents were permitted to remain on their parents' insurance plan until their 26th birthday, and regulations implemented under the Act include dependents that no longer

live with their parents, are not a dependent on a parent's tax return, are no longer a student, or are married.

8.   Insurers are prohibited from dropping policyholders when they get sick.

9.   Insurers will be required to spend 85% of large-group premiums, 80% of small-group premiums, and individual plan premiums on health care or to improve health-care quality, or return the difference to the customer as a rebate.

10. Insurers are prohibited from discriminating against or charging higher rates for any individuals based on pre-existing medical conditions.

11. Insurers are prohibited from establishing annual spending caps.

12. New tax reporting changes come into effect which aims to prevent tax evasion by corporations.

13. All existing health insurance plans must cover approved preventive care and checkups without co-payment.

14. Establish health insurance exchanges, and subsidization of insurance premiums for individuals with income up to 400% of the poverty line, and for single adults.

Cons

1. Creation of task forces on Preventive Services and Community Preventive Services to develop, update, and disseminate evidenced-based recommendations on the use of clinical and community prevention services.

2. The President established a new council within the Department of Health and Human Services, the National Prevention, Health Promotion and Public Health Council, to help begin to develop a National Prevention and Health Promotion Strategy.

3. Annual self-employment and wages of individuals above $200,000 ($250,000 for families) would be subject to an additional tax of 0.5%.

4. Impose a $2000 per employee tax penalty on employers with more than 50 employees who do not offer health insurance to their full-time workers.

5. A new 40% excise tax on high cost insurance plans would be introduced.

6. Impose an annual penalty of $95, or up to 1% of income, whichever is greater, on individuals who do not secure insurance; this would rise to $695, or 2.5% of income, by 2016. This is an

individual limit; families have a limit of $2,085. Exemptions to the fine in cases of financial hardship or religious beliefs are permitted.

7. Provide an advanced, refundable tax credit to provide a government benefit to people even with no tax liability.

8. Health insurance companies would become subject to a new excise tax based on their market share.

9. A new excise tax would go into effect that is applicable to pharmaceutical companies and is based on the market share of the company.

10. Most medical devices would become subject to a 2.3% excise tax collected at the time of purchase.

11. Eliminating the Medicare Part D gap affectionately called the "donut hole".

ACA Amendments

The bill in its original form was amended by the Health Care and Education Reconciliation Act signed on March 30, 2010. The proposed changes were accepted by congress for placing limitations on the bill, as well as expanding certain provisions. The education reform will not be addressed in this review, but the amended bill introduced the following:

1. Increase the tax credits to buy insurance.

2. Eliminates several of the special deals given to senators

3. Lowered the penalty for not buying insurance from $750 to $695.

4. Closed the Medicare Part D "donut hole" by 2020 and gives seniors a rebate of $250.

5. Delayed the implementation on taxing Cadillac health-care plans until 2018.

6. Requires doctors who treat Medicare patients be reimbursed at the full rate.

7. Set up a Medicare tax on the unearned incomes of families that earn more than $250,000 annually.

8. Households below 150% of the federal poverty level would pay 2% to 4% of their income on premiums. Health plans would cover 94% of the cost of benefits.

9. Households with incomes from 150% to 400% of the federal poverty level would pay on a sliding scale from 4% to 9.8% of their income on premiums; the rest would be covered by a government advanced, refundable tax credit. Health plans would cover 70% of the cost of the benefits.

10. Increase the penalty to $2,000 for each full time worker in the company, but would exempt the first 30 employees while calculating the penalty. Increase Medicaid payment rates to primary care doctors to match Medicare payment rates, which are higher, in 2013 and 2014.

11. The federal government would pay all of the costs of expanding Medicaid under the reform until 2016, 95% in 2017, 94% in 2018, 93% in 2019, and 90% thereafter. Some states that already insure childless adults under Medicaid would receive more federal money for covering that group through 2018.

12. Medicare patients would receive a 50% discount on brand-name drugs would begin in 2011. By 2020, the government would pay to provide up to a 75% discount on brand-name and generic drugs, eventually closing the coverage gap.

13. Would extend the ban on lifetime limits and rescission of coverage to all existing health plans within six months after being signed into law.

Financial Impact of the ACA

The Congressional Budget Office (CBO) estimates the Act will reduce the federal deficit by 143 billion dollars in the first decade and by 1.2 trillion dollars in the second decade. There are several views, pro and con, of the ACA, ranging from business commissions to the Medicare and Medicaid service. The changes in the financial picture also affects those who would be able to be insured under the ACAs provisions.

The Act would impose an excise tax on insurance plans with relatively high premiums; and make various other changes to the federal tax code, Medicare, Medicaid, and other programs. The Business Roundtable, an association of CEOs, commissioned a report from the consulting company Hewitt Associates that found that the legislation potentially reduce the rate of future health care cost increases by 15% to 20%. The Office of the Actuary at the Centers for Medicare and Medicaid Services released a report in April 2010 saying the Act would increase the number of Americans with health insurance coverage, but also increased the projected spending by approximately 1% over 10 years.

Public Opinion

In review of the data and statistics concerning the new act, it is clear the provisions of the ACA will leave a profound mark on the economic structure of the nation. The overarching answer as to whether this mark is positive or negative is yet to be seen. Most condemnation and adoration of the bill has been both highly publicized and politicized, so it is up to the people to read the document and understand how it might affect their overall life.

One thing, in my opinion, that has been previously stated is whether the Act is truly healthcare reform or is it health reform through lowering the price of insurance. Healthy People 2010 mentioned the need for access to care being a priority because it crosses socioeconomic and racial lines. However, will the implementation of the ACA going to orchestrate an overhaul of the escalating price of health?

Once again, this answer is yet to be determined because the full effects of the law have yet to be vetted. The fear of change has gripped both sides of the political spectrum without a clear understanding of the Act's provisions. There were several polls on this subject prior to its signing which highlighted the opinions of the Act.

A CNN poll of 1,030 adult Americans found that:

1. 59% opposed the legislation while 39% supported it. Further breakdown showed that 43% opposed the bill because it was too liberal. 13% opposed it because it was not liberal enough.

2. 56% of the respondents in their replies stated the bill gives the government too much involvement in health care; 28% said it gives the government a proper role; and 16% said the government's role would be inadequate.

3. 62% believed the cost associated with the bill would increase the amount of money they personally spend on health care.

4. 37% believed their costs would either remain the same or go down.

5. 70% believed the fiscal implications of the bill would lead to higher deficits; 17% believed there would be no change; and 12% said the deficits would decrease.

A March 22 *USA Today*/Gallup poll of 1,005 adults found that 49% of the respondents viewed the legislation as a good thing or otherwise reacted positively, while about 40% viewed it badly or otherwise reacted negatively.

In response to the public opinion, which have both good and bad points in regards to the merits of the bill, want to see reduced spending in the cost of care while providing assistance to those who cannot afford it. Even now, I have heard from people who have benefitted from being able to purchase insurance through the exchange, and I have heard the horror stories about their insurance premiums increasing exponentially. Using some form of logic to speak on this subject, I thought about another form of mandated insurance that most people do not complain about at all. Let's talk about car insurance.

Health Commodities

What does this matter in a health discussion? How is this even relevant? Is this really an apple to orange comparison? Well I found out through experience that having proof of insurance is the second thing a person is asked for when being stopped for a traffic violation or if you are involved in an accident. You take out insurance because you desire to protect your asset from the possibility of damage, and to have the security of knowing your vehicle can be repaired if it is damaged without question.

Health insurance does the same thing, it protect a very valuable asset from being damaged through wellness exams, by receiving proper medication, and being able to access alternative methods of treatment. It provides the security to know the asset can be repaired without question if damaged. The asset in question is our body, so now the analogy becomes a little clearer as we ask do we love our things more than we love ourselves. Do we cherish our possessions more than our bodies?

I do not believe health insurance should be mandated, but I strongly believe it should be able to be made affordable to every person who desires insurance. However, the overall cost of insurance is too high for people to afford, so they are effectively priced out of a product. The overall merit of the Act itself is in a too close to call stage. It will take some time to reveal the true positives and negatives of the new health mandates.

Health Matters

Like most laws, the conversation about this bill has been wrapped around individuals, politicians, and organizations attempting to score political points and rally their respective bases to action. Health does have political undertones and overtures; however, when does health trump the base political spectrum to transcend talking points and begin a conversation about real change? The answer is not simple, but the people who could benefit the most from the program are the pawns on the political chessboard.

So what does this really mean for people? What does it mean for providers? What does it mean for insurers? What does it mean for the overall health of the country? These are questions no one really wants to answer because it will reveal the need for common sense instead of political correctness and posturing.

The passage of the bill has brought out both advocates and dissenters who argue the pros and cons of the bill through very partisan glasses. In review of the law, it does have some merit, but I always wonder aloud about the growing cost of healthcare and its affordability. Healthcare is not a constitutional right; however, there is a longtime trend of caring for the public welfare of the people.

There is a huge public swell about how healthcare should be administered in this country. It is truly a "free" market where the customer is king, or it is a "privileged" market where those with money can receive better care and benefits? Honestly, it is a combination of both where we are free to choose our providers based on our ability to pay. The Affordable Care Act is supposed to erase this blurred line, but time will be the ultimate judge on whether this becomes a reality.

Political Diversion

In order for this Act to be beneficial to the people it is intended to serve, politicians need to address a fundament gripe most Americans have about our current system; it is not affordable. There are several opponents and proponents concerning the affordability of care, but the common

41

person can truly observe the damage done by not having proper medical care and preventative treatments. The elements of affordability, business buy-in, and consumer protections creates the space for a very innovative and substantive discussion about the state of health in the nation.

The new laws also poses a question to advocate and adversary alike, if this current system is not good, then what should be erected, legislated, and turned into an effective alternative? Here are a few statements concerning the current and future state of the healthcare system:

- "Obamacare is a perfect tool to crush free enterprise and force all Americans into a socialist health care system."

- "America has the best doctors, the best nurses, the best hospitals, the best medical technology, and the best medical breakthrough medicines in the world. There is absolutely no reason we should not have in this country the best health care in the world."

- "Ultimately, health care fails the most basic test. It's not organized around the needs of the patient."

- "I think we can see how blessed we are in America to have access to the kind of health care we do if we are insured, and even if uninsured, how there is a safety net. Now, as to the problem of how much health care costs and how we reform health care ... it is another story altogether."

- "I think the first and principle objective is to repeal Obamacare before it does lasting, fundamental damage to our health care system, to our individual liberty, to the relationship each of us has with his or her doctor."

- "Health is like money, we never have a true idea of its value until we lose it."

There are thousands of quotes and statements that can be applied to argue for and against the Affordable Care Act. In reading some of the statements, it is obvious there are some very strong proponents and opponents to the Act. In short, the sway of public opinion starts from the top and works its way down to the people. However, the groundswell of support often starts at the bottom and fights to rise to the top.

It is the common man's landscape, health, and life versus the corporate giants. It is a fight to develop a system where both can profit, grow and flourish in a wonderful symbiotic relationship. However, the push for health can make it seem to be a little more than a parasitic adventure.

The Future of the Act

The future of the ACA does not rest in the hands of the people, it is solely based on the political landscape of the country. The overall view of the Act has had both positive and negative reviews, so the likelihood of its survival will rest in the hands of our elected officials. I believe there is a fine line between establishing mandates and creating practical solutions because the devil is often lost in the details of the plan.

From a business perspective, do the benefits outweigh the risks? Are the people truly better off with the existing system? Are people more secure in knowing their health is in their hands? Will the existing and future costs of healthcare be the factor that undermines the Act? Will the people be willing to embrace the potential of higher premiums, potential fines, and economic insecurity? The questions and concerns for this Act will be never-ending; however, the most prudent question to ask would be if the needs of the many outweigh the needs of the few. I believe this answer will require soul searching and a true, deep reflection of us as individuals and as a nation. Only time will tell what our response will be to the question.

The World Health Organization defines health as "a state of complete physical, mental, and social well-being and not merely the absence of disease of infirmity." The ability to understand health geography reveals the relationship between this population's center and their environment from a holistic space of packaging, location, and health patterns. The Social Cognitive Theory (SCT) is based on how positive social and personal development occurs in individuals based on their current experience, environment, and personal motivators. Therefore, the application of change through self-efficacy can be causal, but ultimately it is set on a foundation of motivation and action.

The Social Learning Theory (SLT) was based on the premise that an individual's behavior could be changed by either direct participation or direct observation. The SLT kept the same premise of behavioral change, but shifted the focus from being a strictly behavioral observation to garnering a greater sense of self-efficacy based on an individual's desire to change through personal motivation. The existence of these factors kept an environmental perspective upfront, and sought to discover how thinking patterns could be evolved to cause the interactive change being prescribed. The most important factor to consider is understanding the role of self-efficacy through a person's personal beliefs, and how do these beliefs present an avenue for development and change.

Changing the focus

The measure of change stated in the social cognitive theory was not solely based on the individual, but acknowledges there is a collective social nexus from which personal choices are derived. Health behaviors and attitudes can be attributed to environmental factors, and this focus can determine whether positive social change could occur through addressing particular health determinants. The theory could be used to explain the dynamic of social development, cognitive process, and goals of an individual, coupled with the realistic vision of balancing beliefs and behaviors from a cultural context.

Behaviors are often subjective, being attributed to their environment where social interactions occur, which can affect a variety of attitudes towards personal health. The inherent idea between behavior and health is to discover if it is a noted pattern or a random effect, visualizing the direct and indirect impact of health outcomes from an economic and communal viewpoint. The greatest challenge in the growing healthcare environment is to better understand the dynamic of the environment, the person, and the community to foster an attitude of better health for all. The overarching stigma of health, ethics, and public policy have also played an intricate role in fighting and addressing health disparities.

By Any Means Necessary

I don't know is the answer most likely not to be given by people when asked about what they would do to maintain, improve, or receive information that could enrich their health. Health often becomes an afterthought because most believe the old philosophy of I am doing to die from something, so I might as well enjoy myself. Therefore, it is not surprising about the amount of disease found in this country and the strain it places on the healthcare system.

Everyone does not view their health as a priority. How many of us only seek treatment when something occurs? If you answered yes to this question then you are not a part of the solution because your treatment is not preventative, but a reaction to the problem. Our healthcare system is more of reaction treatment system than a preventative one because our habits preclude us from seeking help until our bodies demand we give it attention. In this day and age we have to make priorities about everything because our resources are limited. We have to choose between food, clothing, shelter, and our health. Health often loses because it is expensive to try to live a healthy lifestyle. When I asked a friend about this concept, she stated to me healthy things don't taste good and they cost more. What is more important if I have five dollars? Eat healthy or eat from the dollar menu at a fast food restaurant? The choice is obvious.

Feast or Famine

It would be safe to say our healthcare system has a similar theme when you consider the price for surgical procedures. Families have to choose between their health and their overall survival. Many communities exists in food deserts, where finding fresh, affordable quality foods without an automobile. The government is lobbying for increasing interventions and program development to ease the chronic disease problem; however, they do not address the reality of economic starvation coupled with an improved urban plan to access better food selections.

It may sound difficult, but good health is determined by your zip code. Live in the wrong one and watch your life expectancy drop a few years; at the same time, you could find yourself susceptible to chronic diseases.

Changing Minds

In order to effectively change behaviors, individuals must realize and accept their current health status. This can be challenging because the human will is ingrained to believe as long as a person is breathing then things must be okay. However, in the wider sense of thinking, the health of an individual does carry a mental component, but its focus is often based on the present moment and not future projecting.

Packaging a health message can be extremely difficult because most of it requires a good network, collaborative efforts, and requires getting buy-in from community leaders, who are often seen as the gatekeepers to the community. This also means shifting communication from a more traditional means to one that was once considered an alternative method. Using these methods of communication is needed to reach populations to promote good health and being able to develop essential programs based on their need.

The changing of behaviors and attitudes of person starts with understanding the environment of the individuals and the circumstances that lead to the behavior in question. Promoting health on a community scale starts on the personal level, and using the each one tell one slogan is a good way to promote health. Through practical application of simply telling someone that if this information has helped you, then sharing this news with someone else could arm them with information that could possibly save or extend their lives.

49

Healthy People

The government reviews the health of the nation through the Healthy People Program, which are strategies designed to improve the nation's health by engaging in dialogue about how bad numbers can be reduced and positive indicators increased. We are now under the Health People 2020 banner, but in essence each program reviews various health indicators like teenage pregnancy, suicide, infant mortality, drug use, and chronic diseases to name a few. Health and economics are very much intertwined because a healthy population means there is a stronger and more vibrant workforce, which in turns increases productivity. The Healthy People objectives review trends and sends out these recommendations to the community for a group think-tank effort to combat them.

The Health People Program does not simply remain a government wish list for health, it becomes a community effort to review, strategize, and promote healthy living in the community. It creates new partnerships and networks in populations who might not have ever engaged in fruitful discussions about health. It starts on a high level but is accomplished through a grassroots approach to understand how individual indicators could be revealed to improve health. The sake of good health transcends

50

politics, race, and socioeconomic factors because rich or poor; GED or Ph.D.; or businessman or day laborer, they all have one thing in common, a need to be in optimal health in order to work and be productive.

Call for advocates

Health is in desperate need for advocates who are willing to stand up and not be afraid of the vast political machines that wish to keep it under certain political reins. The adoption of policy is often done by giving oil to the squeaky wheel; however, the need for reform goes beyond simple noise and seeks to find a voice to bring about positive social change. The mentioning of the word "social" in the political world automatically denotes paying homage to a particular party and determining whether the rich or poor would benefit from the program.

Social change in this narrative refers to the ability for a nation to not simply throw money at a problem, but to instinctively and empathically collaborate to ascertain advantageous solutions to a growing problem. It is true that our health infrastructure is bursting at the seams and there does not appear to be a light at the end of the proverbial tunnel. The question for health advocates is to appeal for the call for reform to not be heavy handed on one side or the other.

The call for advocacy reaches out to community leaders and other heads of civic and service organizations to stand up and be a voice of reason at a time where it appears saner heads cannot prevail. The development of policy should not be left in the hands of special interest, PACS, Super PACS, and lobbyist; it should be done with the voice of the people it intends to impact the most. However, most laws and policies formed in our country are performed in a vacuum, accepting the opinions of a small number of like-minded constituents to legislate decisions for society at large.

Chapter 5: The Future of Health

The future of health in the United States is an undiscovered country because we understand and acknowledge the premise of healthcare, but disagree on the right path to reach a logical conclusion to solve the paradigm. The burden of this responsibility does not solely lie with our politicians, but with every citizen who is determined to not let the status quo be our silent death. As in the previous chapter that spoke about politics, our health should not be acquainted to the proverbial carrot on a stick; however, any discussion should be transformative and thought provoking in nature.

Our nation is getting older, getting grayer, and will have an influx of veterans with a variety of health concerns. At the same time, the general population is not improving their eating habits, not exercising, and we are becoming over dependent on technology. I am not saying technology is bad, but how many children still go outside and play for least 30 minutes in the sun versus spending hours on video games? How many kids still ride bikes? How many of us exercise for at least 15-20 minutes a day? Our sedimentary lifestyles will one day lead to our demise.

An anonymous author once said, "Just because you're not sick doesn't mean you're healthy." This is the realism we face as a nation. The declining health of America is a real epidemic that must be taken into consideration if we plan to extend our lives on this planet and to fulfill our many wishes and dreams for both ourselves and our children. The decline does not mean our science and technology is waning, it means health is not the number one priority of the country.

The Politics of Health

There is an iron triangle in health that consists of producers, consumers, and legislators. One side of the triangle is dependent upon the other; however, the size and length of each leg of the triangle is what often makes a difference in passing policies. The word "health" does not appear in the constitution but there is a mention of providing for the general welfare. It is here were we find the basis of legal arguments for and against the healthcare system in this country.

The ability to change a system from the inside requires considerable courage because most legislation has been buffeted by special interest groups who desire to have "favorable" legislation passed. This bridge of healthcare is supported by the towers of action and trust, while it is wired by the meanings or actual words embedded in the legislation. However, most laws are either given to the highest bidder or is a knee-jerk reaction to an event, so the crafting of promising bills are left to the mercy of the party who resides in the seat of power.

Programs, People, or Productivity

The fight for insurance is not about anti-equality, it is about the power to control, shape, mold, or break people's lives. This is often performed through inaction or by producing ineffective programs. It is no secret the healthcare question has resurfaced and what we are seeing is not one to be proud of in any way, shape, or form.

The problem is not medicine, it is the skyrocketing costs, the lack of access, and not enough messages of prevention. We often don't like to talk about issues that demand soul-searching answers. We don't like to discuss issues that make us question our own moral deficiencies, over judgmental opinions, and lack of empathy.

In some ways, we think like Charles Darwin's evolutionary theory of survival of the fittest. There is no way our thinking could be this base; however, I would like to present compelling evidence to make us think differently. Let the market determine how to price insurance; the government should not be in the insurance business, leave it to the companies; businesses reduce employee hours to avoid offering insurance;

insurance rates increase; deductibles increase; socialism, death panels, long lines, extended suffering, month long appointments, and other phrases for or against our current system of care.

The nation's health has become a pawn in the political game of chess. Politicians, on both side of aisle, pander and pull on the heartstrings of people to see their point. We observe other nations and mock them because they have a different system and culture of dealing with one another.

However, our current system of capitalism cannot be compared to their standard. Not disagreeing or agreeing; however, I do see the positives and negatives of working together in this kind of system. Instead of putting our heads together, talking with common folk, researching the idea, and creating public groundswell, we are quite content to call each other names and invoke unproven fears because this is the best way to get our point across instead of having a logical discussion on solving our problems.

Providing Service

A unique function of the healthcare system is understanding all the variables: external environment, mission statements, strategic plans, and organizational networks to name a few. You also have to review the providers, such as insurance carriers, primary care providers, and drug companies. Everything has a price that is paid by the consumer; however, how fair is the price in comparison to other countries. For example, in 2007, a knee replacement in the United States cost $14,946. This is compared to $14,608 in Australia; $12,424 in France; $10,438 in Sweden; $10, 011 in the Netherlands; $9,910 in Canada; and $9,931 in Finland.

We are faced with a severe burden of chronic diseases which will tax our already bulging system to its breaking point. Experts predict the future costs of treating these diseases will cost in the excess of 1 trillion dollars. This experiment in human health does not take this data into consideration because our social consciousness is not keeping up with the ills of our society. The fundamental issue is not why people's health have reached disparaging numbers, but how do economic factors play an intricate role in the rise of the numbers.

Low income is a mirror of lower education, lower earning potential, having to make decisions based on finances, not being able to afford healthy foods, not able to engage in external functions, and increases alcohol and drug dependency. Yes, there are services and "safety nets" for this segment of the population, but our goal should not be to simply catch people who fall, but to find ways to prevent them from falling. Packaging good health and healthy practices is beneficial to everyone, and the insurance conversation is an excellent commencement to ensure we do not simply provide insurance but to install an educational component for positive reinforcement about maintaining good health.

Getting to Yes

Getting legislation passed sometimes has to deal with mastering the art of negotiation. How to get to yes is a pragmatic question because it requires both sides involved to determine interest and alternatives and identify potential options in order to move forward. The issue becomes quite interesting when determining whose best interest is being considered in regards to the complexities of the bill.

Most laws are passed in a winner takes all scenario, where controversial bills are often not sent for a vote unless there is a solid majority backing the bill. Health and healthcare has been very unsettling because regular people suffer while politicians engage in pandering and grandstanding. Leaders from the health sector are needed to provide their knowledge, skills, and expertise to assist in crafting legislation with the understanding not everyone is going to get everything they desire.

For most in the legislative branch of government, the decision-making process can be a make or break type of deal. However, the issue moving in the undercurrent is how to craft a bill that covers what the majority of country desires and maintain their fiscal responsibility? This is where the conflict arises and resolving the issue requires a great deal of patience. The average citizen is looking for stability, good rate, good coverage, and a low deductible for services.

The outcomes for such laws look at social, behavioral, and organizational evolution, as well as possible changes in programs that will require adjustments to the evaluation process. The foundation of health lies in communication and the ability to engage in open dialogue about the strengths, weaknesses, opportunities, and threats that can be addressed and mitigated to the best of every party's ability.

Communicating health concerns can be a complicated issue because the ability to get facts, truth, and other relevant data can be stifled or simply unheard because of its source. The ability to communicate risk could result in laying out a diagram of how the nation's health is affected by day to day politics could be a complicated issue. However, the ability to enter into dialogue could reveal the space between health and healthcare to solve this growing crisis.

Getting the Oil

An old adage says the squeaky wheel gets the oil. Our current healthcare system is broken and squeaking loud, but it is not getting the oil it requires to move the gears of change. Usually, this occurs because our politicians are trapped between money and principle, and money often wins out because they need the financial support to maintain future campaign plans and other political ventures.

The gears of change want to move; however, the ability to compromise of issues is a moot point in today's political climate. Decisions are based on a think tank mentality instead of actively moving according to one's conscious. It would not be logical to assume they are unaware of the problems we face as a nation in regard to health and insurance, but will standing for principle mean turning their back on a party's political platform?

Whether this position is in theory or in practice, our current situation is going nowhere fast and now is the time for action. In review of quality indicators and other methods of analysis, our country is getting older and sicker by the day. Community health departments and other governmental agencies have spoken out about the afflictions of the community and how this ties into becoming a national epidemic.

60

However, the legislators must move with them in order to have the interventions and programs necessary for true change.

What's Next?

The 21st century in America will indeed be very interesting. Many of the healthcare laws we have on the books will be challenged even more. The political side of the equation has legislators choosing to either support or assault the existing laws. The human side of the equation want politicians to review the crumbling infrastructure of our system and find ways to fix it.

The health battle has morphed from a personal affair to a financial decision. How much are you worth? What risks do you bring to the table? Is there a logical reason to not offer health insurance? These are the common sense questions many people have but their attention is turned to the people making the most noise. No law is perfect, no idea is the best; however, having some direction is better than having none at all.

The message goes beyond simply having insurance, it is ensuring people have places to walk, exercise, and buy healthy foods at an affordable price. It is about having supermarkets that offer a variety of food choices besides being a community loaded down with fast food restaurants. Food deserts do exist in this day and age, but we worry more about your health by county and zip code. It is not rocket science to understand how health conditions vary according to socioeconomic indicators. It is equally disturbing to see how little information reaches their hands in the community to educate and assist them to move forward to have better health.

The plight of the community lies in the extended hand of the government, who has had a role in the creation of generational poverty and dependency. The hidden discussion of real empowerment is lost behind the smokescreens and mirrors by those who seek for the masses to remain ignorant to the real issues and facts surrounding them. People are being lead like sheep off a cliff because we refuse to wake up and see our reality for what it is.

It reminds me of the Matrix where Neo had to take either the red or blue pill. One would leave him connected to the machines and the other would free him to face the horror of a post-apocalyptic reality. Many people are willing to live in a false sense of reality, not understanding the years of life and vitality being lost due to lacking the necessary information required to make informed health decisions.

From a community health standpoint, there is a need to have more knowledgeable people to develop and sustain a more reflective, health conscious community. The creation of external materials could be used to further this cause, understanding not everyone will take advantage of the opportunities. However, it is successful if one person can be positively affected by the programs and provide informational materials specifically designed to improve their personal health.

Relationship Building

The future of nation's health is predicated upon positive collaborations and networking, understanding our life expectancy and other indicators will not improve unless all hands are on deck of the ship called health and are rowing in the same direction. Our current health directives and programs are very polarizing because we are not truly considering the needs of the people. In this narrative the ability to save and assist everyone may not be possible, but our neighboring and peer countries continue to show us that different programs can be successfully implemented. We must now make a choice to decide if we are for the greater good or for the greater few.

The passage of the ACA could be considered a step in the right direction to open up constructive dialogue about the future of health and healthcare in this country. The ever swinging pendulum of health is feeling more like a guillotine, with the heads of many falling underneath the weight of its sharp blade. Whether we plan for overhauling the "universal coverage" or the "single payer plans", the goal will remain the same, how to effectively cover the nation's citizens without breaking their backs in order to achieve the outcomes desired by officials.

Health, an undiscovered country, is going to be a topic of conversation for the next generation because our country is getting grayer with the baby boomers now reaching the age of retirement and the childbirth rates are slowing. We must now make decisions to protect the offspring of the "greatest generation". We must now begin to focus on "generation x" and the "millennials" who will be charged with carrying this extreme mantle of leadership and responsibility. Time will reveal what the ending to this narrative will be; either good for some, bad for others; good for all; or bad all around.

Maybe we should heed the advice of a popular science fiction alien who once said the needs of many outweigh the needs of the few…

ABOUT THE AUTHOR

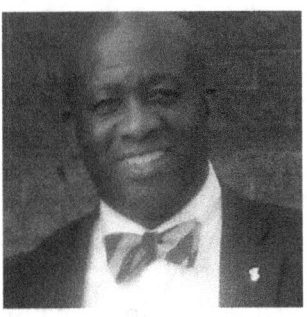

Keith E. Lindsey, Ph.D., author of "The Twelve Experiences",
has performed several speaking engagements about health and
how it affects various populations and age groups. He also talks
about chronic diseases, finances, and community engagement to
promote advocacy.

Keith is the Owner of The Lindsey Group, an organization that
focuses on education, health, finances, and community advocacy.

Keith grew up in New York City, but now resides in Tennessee.
In his spare time, Keith enjoys music, electronics, reading, and
writing, and sports.